Makeup
Magic

Toni Thomas

DEDICATION

For every self-assured woman who wants to
stand out from the crowd and love themselves
for who they are. Go confidently in your
journey to enhance the beauty of you.

CONTENTS

ACKNOWLEDGMENTS

To my talented friend, beauty photographer Keisha Garrett, without her photography skills I would not be able to share my makeup knowledge with you. Her pictures show what only I can explain in words.

Makeup Confidence

It begins and ends with you.

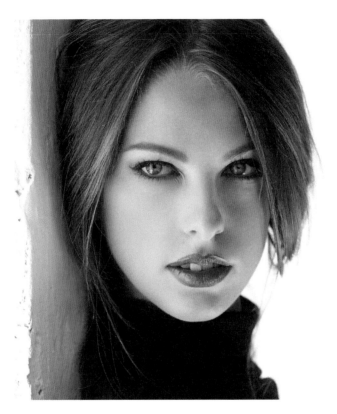

No face is perfect and as much as we would like
to have the qualities we admire in others we are
each of us individuals and that is what makes
us so special and unique, the truth is someone
else is admiring those same qualities about

you. Our uniqueness is what gives us our beauty, it is in these differences that we find our strengths, those that give us the confidence to live in our own skin.

Makeup is all about enhancing our own personal uniqueness and appreciating those qualities we want to improve upon. As much as we hear just love the woman you are, most women do not take this to heart and try to blend in with the masses. But to achieve self-confidence we need to cherish our faces for what they are and enhance the features we know are our best assets.

Self-assured women enhance their imperfections, they embrace them and even applaud them. They know where their strengths lie, where they can improve and when to adjust them to get the results they want. Trying to look perfect or look like someone else just takes away from your originality and blends you into the crowd. A self-assured woman wants to stand out from the crowd and love themselves for who they are and how they look. Having a makeup plan to enhance your features is the first step in acquiring makeup confidence.

Makeup Plan

The makeup plan starts with a truth session with yourself. What are you willing to do each day and how much time can you commit to your makeup routine. Next, you need to assess what your skin or seek a professional assessment from a trained makeup or skincare professional. They will help you understand your skin tone and the makeup products that will look best on you, they will help you assess your skin type to determine the best products to use and lastly, if they are good at what they do they will show you how to properly apply the products you will be using.

If you have worked with a professional makeup artist before and you are comfortable they can achieve the look you want, by all means have your makeup done by the pro. But if that isn't the case there are a few ways you can achieve a flawless and glowing makeup application doing it yourself and getting the professional results you are looking for.

Makeup never looked so good or was so easy to achieve when done by a woman who has learned the skills to do flawless makeup on herself.

Your desire to have a beautiful makeup application starts with gaining confidence in your makeup skills and knowing what's truly important when it comes to the presentation of your makeup. The key to makeup success will require practicing what you learn, understanding how to apply makeup, using the right tools, and gaining the knowledge about quality makeup and which colors best suit you.

Makeup

Makeup is as special as you are, no two women are alike, no two faces are alike and no makeup application is the same for everyone. You are a confident woman and should have a vision for your makeup look and you deserve to look exactly as you choose. Your makeup look should require a little research on your part. Go out and scout out certain makeup looks online. Get familiar with what you find attractive and what you know would be your preferred look. Doing your research is essential to gaining your makeup confidence and to achieve the look you want.

With so many makeup application options how can you achieve the right look for you?

The great thing about makeup is there are no rules, makeup is a creative process that lets the person who is applying the makeup be as original and unique as they choose to be or as structured as is necessary, but when it comes to your daily makeup application there are a few guidelines to follow.

- A perfectly matched foundation is essential to a successful makeup application, it should be an exact match to your skin tone and look dewy once applied.

- A three-color eye shadow application with a less is more approach will bring your face forward showcasing your eyes, giving depth and dimension to your everyday look.

- Perfectly applied blush using a two color application will give you lasting results that will carry you through the day and into the evening.

- Subtle contouring can give you an instant facelift and project a confident you.

- Your highlighter will bring a radiant glow to your face creating a luminous look.

- Filling in your brows with a brow product gives your face structure.

- Applying a lip color even if it's just a gloss is very important

- Using at least one coat of mascara will enhance any makeup look.

Makeup Balance

Your makeup needs to reflect not only your personality and enhance your own inner beauty but it will also need to highlight your best features. If you are doing an everyday makeup look you will want it to be subtle and just enough to give your face and features a little life.

A workday look is meant to brighten your cheeks, lips, and eyes to bring life to your face and overcome the harsh overhead lights at the office.

A weekend look should be natural and carefree, using just a few products to give you a glowing look without looking overdone or overly made up. The weekends are all about fun and enjoying your life, this is truly where less is more will work for you.

An evening look should be more bold with deeper tones and a bit heavier application, this will enhance your features even in low light. Evening makeup is all about romance, sophistication and even a little drama.

Whatever your makeup needs you will find that following a 10 step makeup routine will work for any occasion.

Ethereal Beauty

For evening makeup you want to portray ethereal beauty that sets the stage for the most romantic and memorable night of your life, this is your chance to try new makeup looks that will not enhance your inner and outer beauty. Your makeup should project a healthy beautiful extension of you and evening makeup is the perfect opportunity to boost your beautiful features and present a radiant woman who is confident, comfortable and ready to take on the world.

Your makeup needs to be as flawless as possible and to achieve this you need to have makeup confidence, this means you will know how to apply your makeup so it appears as if it were applied by a professional. This means perfectly matched foundation and makeup in the right hues and tones that goes on smooth and are evenly applied over the entire face, chin, neck and chest using a blending technique that gives the appearance of airbrush makeup without using an airbrush.

This guide is going to show you how to get that airbrushed look as well as many other tips, tricks, and secrets to achieving that flawless wedding day makeup application.

In the following sections, you are going to learn our exclusive 10-step makeup application that will ensure you are the most beautiful you. If you follow the steps and practice each application using the rights tools and products you will have the makeup confidence to create the most beautiful you any day or night. Makeup confidence starts with understanding the three key elements in makeup, even the most confident makeup artist will tell you she had to practice her skills on many faces before perfecting her techniques. As a makeup artist, she has spent countless hours practicing her techniques to achieve the skills she has learned to apply flawless and well executed makeup. A makeup artist has many assets but her number one asset is the brushes she uses to apply makeup on her clients. To achieve makeup success she must use high-quality makeup applied with quality brushes using a blending technique that gives a flawless finish. Although makeup has no rules there are a few simple techniques in the makeup application that you will need to follow to give you the results you are looking for as you build your knowledge base and gain the confidence required to have success in your makeup application.

Key Elements in Makeup

Practice: Each day you will need to practice all the steps or certain application aspects that you may struggle with to give you the advantage of a flawless finish. Practicing will, in turn, give you the makeup confidence you need for a successful makeup application. Once you begin practicing every day you will be surprised at how many compliments you will receive about how beautiful and glowing you look, thus ensuring your makeup confidence even more.

Tools: Your tools and brushes will be an important aspect of your makeup application and in all the makeup you will do for the rest of your life. Test your new brushes, do they feel good in your hand, do they put down the product the way they were designed, are they easy to maneuver in your hand, and are the bristles held firmly in the ferrule of the brush and not coming off on your face? If so then you have found the perfect brushes for you.

Makeup & Blending: Sounds so simple right? Apply the makeup and then blend it all in! The truth is choosing the right makeup is going to be a very important step in your makeup application success. Makeup is a multi-billion dollar industry and this means that you the consumer have many choices. Some makeup is good, some makeup not so good but most cosmetics are somewhere in the middle. It doesn't really matter what makeup brand you choose, just choose a quality brand that works well with your skin, matches your skin tone and isn't harmful to your skin. There is nothing worse than bad makeup that is also harmful to you and your skin. So take your time, get to know what works best for you and what products you like to use. Get familiar with makeup products, go to cosmetic counters and get samples, if your friends are selling a makeup or skincare brand ask for samples.

Skincare Secrets
True beauty lies in well loved skin.

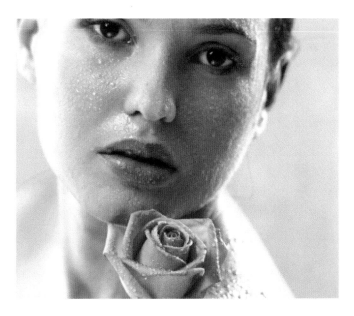

Did you know you can only feed your skin from within? Most topical beauty products and their applications do not nourish our skin; they were designed to protect and maintain our skin. So it is up to each of us to maintain a balanced diet while drinking our recommended daily amount of pure water. These elements are the most precious gifts we can give our skin and our bodies. A lack of water is the principal cause of daytime fatigue, under eye bags and poor skin conditions. Good skincare, as well as a well-balanced diet, are the first steps in a having a great makeup application, it will be up to you to start your skincare routine as soon as possible and stick to it forever.

As a woman who wants to have a flawless face, it is your responsibility to prepare your skin for before your makeup application and maintain healthy vibrant skin throughout your lifetime. Proper skincare is important since the skin is the canvas you will lay your makeup upon and it needs to be healthy, plump and free of skin issues. With that in mind remember the secret to healthy, beautiful, and glowing skin is drinking your daily recommend amount of water to maintain that healthy glow.

Do you know the recommended daily amount of water you need?

Use a simple water rule to calculate your needed water intake.

Divide your body weight by 16 and the resulting number is the recommended daily amount of water you need to consume every day. (Example: 125 lbs. divided by 16 equals = 7.8 glasses of water daily)

The skin is made up of 70% water and needs as

much hydration as possible to keep it looking its optimal best. Studies show that 75% of the US population is dehydrated and many Women are functioning in a state of chronic dehydration resulting in a loss of focus, slower brain function, and poor skin. With this knowledge, it is easy to see why many women have skin issues that give the appearance of fine lines, bags under the eyes and that less than a healthy glow we are seeking. Solving some skin issues could be as easy as drinking plenty of water and seeking the advice of a skincare professional.

Skincare Professional

When is it time to seek the help of a skincare professional?

For many women seeking the help of a skincare specialist is as easy as making an appointment with a local esthetician at a skin salon or day spa, for other women with chronic skin issues you might need to seek a more advanced skincare specialist or dermatologist. No matter what route you choose we recommend seeking the advice of a skincare professional to at least help you get started on the skincare routine suited for your skin and your skin type. Your first step could be as simple as making an appointment for a facial at your local spa or salon, get an analysis of your skin and let an expert recommend the best skincare routine based on the skin analysis you receive.

If we can only feed the body and skin from within what is the point of good skincare? Why should we use quality skincare and not just soap and water? According to Kate Tart, the lead esthetician for Derma E, "Applying your skin care products in the proper order ensures that your skin receives the full benefits of each product." For example, if you applied a cream-based moisturizer followed by a serum, the cream's emolliency would prevent the serum from reaching the skin. Many moisturizers also contain water, and if you apply a moisturizer over a sunscreen, you would in effect be watering down your sunscreen and diluting its effectiveness. Aside from the order of application it's also important to consider the time it takes for your skin to absorb your products.

Did you know that benzoyl peroxide, which is commonly found in acne-treatment regimens, has a one-to three-hour activation time, so any cream or lotion that comes in contact with it before it has completed its work will likely inhibit the active ingredient from working properly?

Skincare is not the only thing you should consider in your skincare routine, you should also be using moisturizers and body lotions that have SPF protection. Applying an SPF sunscreen is necessary not only for long-term healthy and beautiful skin but for short term as well. SPF or sun protection factor comes in various sun blocking abilities but even the highest level SPF must be re-applied every 2-3 hours to be effective. According to Web MD, an SPF 15 product blocks about 94% of UVB rays; an SPF 30 product blocks 97% of UVB rays; and an SPF 45 product blocks about 98% of rays. Sunscreens with higher SPF ratings block slightly more UVB rays, but none offers 100% protection and as we said before you should be reapplying your SPF every 2-3 hours to maintain protection.

Note that some photographers discourage the application of SPF products on the day of a photo shoot, so if you do your makeup for a professional photo shoot you should skip the SPF. SPF is known to cause what photographers call flash-backs that make you look pale and can give the face dusty white cast in photos. So in this one instance put away the SPF and just use a good moisturizer.

You are in charge of your skin, it is up to you to keep it as healthy as possible.

The Skincare Routine

Your skincare routine is a very important element when trying to achieve a flawless makeup application. How your skin is functioning will have an impact on your appearance, skincare is a lifestyle decision and should be a part of your everyday routine. If you don't currently have a routine it is a good idea to start looking at skincare products and what you should be using.

A solid skincare routine should start immediately and if you don't know what that means then visit your local esthetician or cosmetics counter to get started on the products that will work well with your skin type. I recommend consulting a professional for a skincare analysis and a facial to jump-start your healthy skincare routine, these professionals are trained to get you started on a healthy skincare routine that will get you the right products suited for your skin and a structured regimen to get your skin functioning properly. Let the professional guide you on your skincare routine and listen to their recommendations, they are the pros and have been trained to assist you in achieving your most healthy skin. Water is essential to luminous and glowing skin but even more important is a healthy diet filled with fresh fruits, vegetables, plant proteins, and lean cuts of meat and fish. It is up to you to avoid foods that can cause skin irritations and outbreaks, so choose to love your skin and give it the nutrients it will need to flourish. Beauty begins with healthy skin and healthy skin begins with a balanced diet and lifestyle. It's time to become your skins best friend.

- *Eat Right*
- *Exercise regularly*
- *Sleep 8-9 hours per night*
- *Restrict sun exposure*
- *Avoid pollutants and smoke*
- *Don't over indulge in alcohol*
- *Minimize stress in your life*

These are only a few steps to take in your skincare routine. As we said before it is always a good idea to consult with an esthetician or dermatologist and get a skincare consultation before starting your skincare routine. These professionals can guide you in the right direction with the best products to use and help you get an understanding of your skin and what will be required to maintain it and keep it in optimal condition.

Few people have perfect skin, in fact, no one is immune to skin issues and skin conditions, there are just too many factors that can affect the balance of our delicate skin. Our skin is not only affected by what we ingest into our system but even the air around us can cause skin issues. So it will be up to you to get familiar with your skin and become your skin's best friend, only then can you have your best skin ever.

Listen to what your skin is telling you, track your skins progress with a journal, and try to get a deep understanding of how your skin wants to be treated. Even sensitive and troubled skin can be transformed into a glowing canvas for you to work with as you move into your daily makeup routine.

Understanding Your Skin Type

After washing your face it's?

- *Tight and a little stretched - Dry*
- *Clean, but shiny within 20min - Oily*
- *In good condition - Normal*
- *Shiny in the "T" zone - Mixed*
- *A little red and stings - Sensitive*

When you don't use lotions your skin is?

- *Rough and scaly. - Dry*
- *Greasy, shiny - Oily*
- *Same as the previous day - Normal*
- *Shiny on the forehead - Mixed*
- *Redness on cheeks - Sensitive*

The skin is the largest organ in our bodies and consists of 70% water so getting familiar with your skin and your skin type is an important part of getting to know more about yourself and understanding how you can care for your skin. Knowing how your skin reacts to products, environment and even to changes in diet as well as activity is key to learning how to care for your most precious commodity.

Therefore getting a good understanding of your

skin type is one of the first steps in your skincare routine. It will be up to you to seek guidance from a skincare specialist who can guide you to the right products and who will give you a skincare roadmap to follow.

This roadmap should be a part of your daily routine for at least six weeks leading up to any big event and healthy looking skin for life.

A Youthful Glow

The skin is our protective barrier against harmful agents such as bacteria, chemicals, ultraviolet rays, pollutants and even water absorption. It is made up of 70% water and it is your greatest asset, so to keep it beautiful it is up to you to protect and nourish it.

Your skin type can be easily determined with a quick assessment and your skincare routine will be based on your skin type and the current condition of your skin. Whatever your skin type there are three basic things to remember to keep it looking youthful and healthy.

- *Clean it daily and always remove all makeup, try using the double cleanse method.*

- *Moisturize and care for your skin with*

products that suit your skin needs.

- *Protect your skin from external elements like the sun, smoke, wind, air conditioning, and all elements that are harmful to your skin.*

A youthful glow no matter what your age can be achieved by making your skin and your skincare routine a top priority. This means planning to be committed to your skincare routine and skincare diet for up to six months prior to your wedding day. Once you have established your skincare routine and diet it will just become a part of your everyday routine.

Your skin is going to last you a lifetime and needs you to care for it as you would a newborn baby, with love, tenderness, and great kindness.

The saying, "love the skin you're in" is a truth most of us can't ignore.

Take the time to understand your skin type and give it the love it needs to give you that youthful and timeless glow. Your skin and your Selfies will love you for it.

Maintaining a youthful glow is easy if you take

the time to love your skin from within. You must also protect it with the right products that will nurture it on the outside and keep it soft and supple and safe from harmful UV rays and pollutants.

Makeup Magic

Your guide to flawless makeup.

Step 1: Primer

The most important step to achieving a lasting daytime makeup look is using a quality primer. Your primer needs to be lightweight and applies easily to the face, neck, and the lids of the eyes. Your primer has two objectives, to keep your makeup in place all day and to minimize the appearance of fine lines and large pores. Your primer will act as a skin sealer keeping your makeup in place all day and concealing those little face flaws no one else needs to see.

Primer is essential to your makeup look and getting the right primer for your skin type will prove to be one of the most important steps in your 10-step makeup application.

- Apply primer over the face and neck.
- Apply eye primer to the lids of the eyes.
- Wait 5 min before applying makeup.

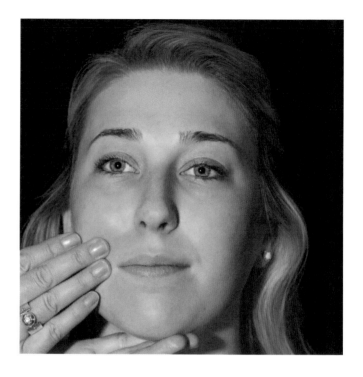

The first step of your makeup application should always be a primer, even when you are only going for a light and airy weekend look. Using a primer will keep your makeup in place all day giving you a polished look even when you are choosing to wear very little makeup. I encourage my clients to use a tinted primer that evens out their skin and can keep even a tinted moisturizer in place all day long.

Step 2: Correct and Conceal

Concealers and correctors are your secret weapon in makeup and help to correct and conceal those tiny flaws on your face. They are essential to a flawless finish.

Correctors are exactly what they claim to be and they are necessary to erase those tiny flaws on your face that can show through your makeup if not taken care of before your foundation is applied. A corrector is used to cover acne spots, scars, and redness on the face or purple hues that often appear under our eyes or on our eyelids. Your corrector colors are usually green, yellow or peach. Green is used to hide red spots from acne. Yellow is used to correct purple hues under the eyes or on the eyelids and pink or peach colored corrector can be used on scars or to neutralize discoloration.

Concealers are more to brighten your face and to cover the correctors you have just applied. I recommend you apply your concealer after you have applied your foundation but you choose the time to apply that best suits your needs.

- Apply a beige or yellow concealer one color lighter than your skin tone under the eyes.
- Create a V shape that runs from under your eye down to the top of your cheek and blend it with upward and outward strokes to the outer corner of your eye.
- Conceal any discoloration.

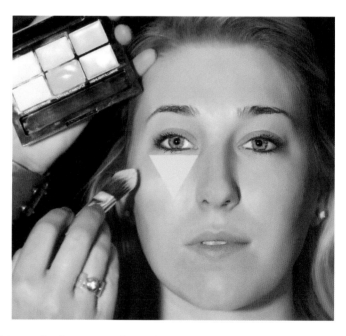

This technique needs to be blended well and must not appear harsh in its finished state.

Learning how to use correctors and concealers will be essential in your makeup routine and once applied they should be blended well on the outer edges of the application. Correcting and concealing takes practice and patience and an understanding of the flaws you want to hide and the areas of the face you want to enhance, this will be crucial to creating a flawless look.

Understating what your corrector palette can do will give you more confidence when you are trying to hide those pesky little flaws on your face.

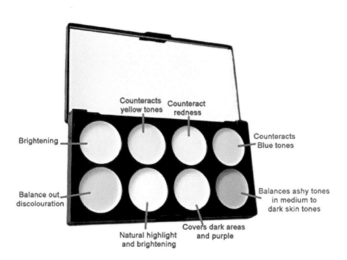

Brightening

Counteracts yellow tones

Counteract redness

Counteracts Blue tones

Balance out discolouration

Natural highlight and brightening

Covers dark areas and purple

Balances ashy tones in medium to dark skin tones

Step 3: Foundation

Finding the correct color and consistency of foundation is a vital step in your makeup application. You want a foundation that is the exact color of your skin tone and at the same time has the right consistency to cover your flaws. You should strip-test every foundation you buy.

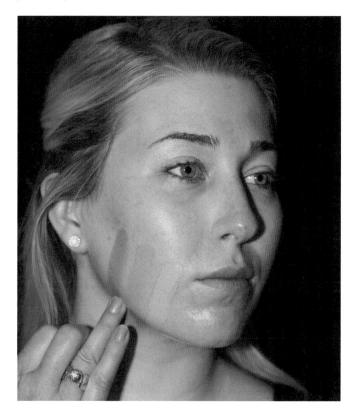

Strip Test

One of the first steps in foundation is finding the right color for your skin. This is a step you will want to make sure you do not skip. Your foundation should be an exact match of your skin and blend seamlessly into your chin and neck. Make sure to do a foundation strip test. Our model has three stripes on her face and one is almost invisible.

Applying Foundation

- Apply foundation to your face using your fingertips covering all areas of the face, this technique warms the product and makes it easy to apply.

- Once you have covered your face, neck and chin use a stiff flat brush to gently blend the product over the entire face, and down the neck giving it an airbrushed finished.

- Check that you have blended well into the sides of the face, the chin and the neck so there are no harsh lines of demarcation.

- Give a final check to make sure your finish is flawless.

5 Rules of Foundation

Can you get a perfect and flawless makeup foundation? Can you really achieve flawless looking skin and still look like you're wearing nothing at all? With a few simple rules to follow you can get the flawless foundation you are looking for.

Five simple rules of foundation and you will get the flawless results you are looking for.

1. Choose the right foundation product.
2. Know what product works best with your skin type (mineral powder foundations, liquid foundations, cream foundations).
3. Choose the correct color.
4. Apply with fingers then use the brush blending technique.
5. Set with a spray or setting powder.

Remember with these simple rules to follow you can get the flawless finished foundation look that will give your skin just the right coverage without hiding your beautiful features.

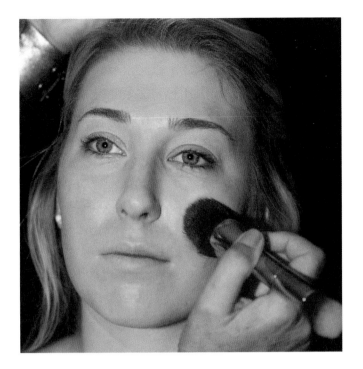

Foundation Options

Powder: Usually a mineral foundation that gives full coverage and works well with oily and youthful skin.

Liquid: Usually leaves a dewy finish that can give you full coverage or a more translucent coverage depending on it's consistency and the application it was designed for. It is perfect for dry skin and older skin.

Cream: A perfect option for giving full coverage to problem skin, cream foundations have a thicker consistency and go on like a liquid and are best applied with beauty blenders or sponges, but remember to use your foundation brush to blend in the hairline and under the chin and neck to give an airbrushed finish.

Flawless

Your foundation will be the most important aspect of your flawless look and it will be your responsibly to make sure you have the right foundation for your skin type and the right foundation color for your skin tone.

The price of your foundation is not as important as how it works with your skin. Foundation prices range drastically from product to product but the reality is, your foundation needs to feel lightweight on your skin, be an exact match to your skin tone and work well with your skin type. If you need assistance with your foundation choice take the time to speak with a professional and get a color match consultation with a pro makeup artist or skincare specialist.

Step 4: Setting Powders

Setting your concealer and foundation is an important step in your makeup application and one you don't want to miss. Use a quality translucent powder or a yellow toned translucent powder on your face and neck to give you a shine-free look that will ensure when your photos arrive your face will have a perfect finish. Setting your foundation can make or break the longevity of your makeup application.

- Use a large puffy brush.

- Choose a quality setting powered that is translucent or yellow toned.

- Be very sparing with your setting powder you don't want your makeup to look caked.

If you have mature skin I suggest not using any powder on your face, powders tend to settle in fine lines and is not a kind product for aging skin.

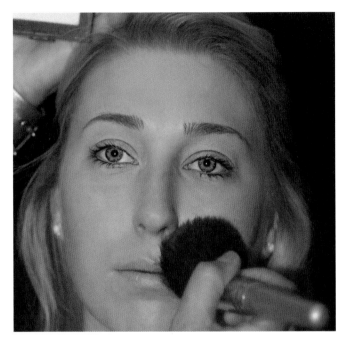

Setting powders come in a wide variety of shades and can come in a compact or loose state. Your setting powder should feel lightweight on your skin and maintain your flawless foundation look. Take the time to research the right setting powder for you and if in doubt that a setting powder is right for you stick to a setting spray that you can use at the end of your makeup application.

Step 5: Contour & Bronze

Everyday makeup is not about heavy contouring or loads of bronzer, it's an opportunity to enhance your best features by giving depth and dimension as well as a natural lift to your face. The same applies to using a bronzer which gives your skin a kiss of sun. Your contour color should be two shades darker than your natural skin tone but not to dark that it will make your face look sculpted, dirty and un-natural.

Contouring

Your cheek contour should not come in further than the outer corner of your eye. Use your contour brush and check where your contour should end.

- Use a contour shade just a bit darker than your skin tone and apply just below each cheek bone, sweeping out toward the hair.

- If necessary on a large forehead contour along the hairline to slim the face.

- Slim down a large chin by placing a fine

dust of contour around the chin enhancing the end of the chin bone.

- If you feel like you need to slim down a sagging chin area, use your contour just under the jawline giving the illusion of shadow to mask a sagging chin area.

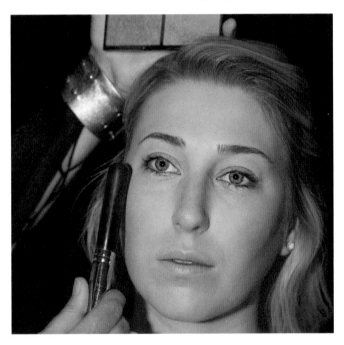

Bronzing

Your secret gift of man made sun.

- Apply bronzer to the chest area if you are wearing a strapless or low cut gown. Be sure to not over do it with your bronzer and choose a shade that brightens not a shade that can make your skin look dirty.

- Apply to the forehead and on the cheeks or anywhere that the sunlight would hit on the face or anywhere that needs a kiss of sun. Do not overdo the bronzer it can quickly darken the face and neck.

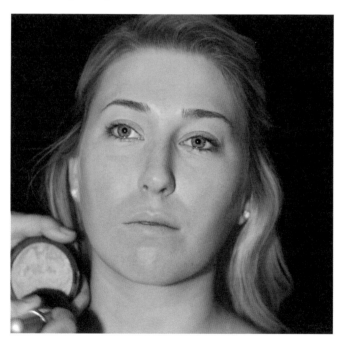

Step 6: Blush

For a fresh and luminous glow use a two-step blush application that will give your face the perfect glow and perk up your skin. Blush when applied correctly wakes the face up and adds warmth. It is applied with a puff brush or blush brush and if done correctly will enhance your features. Blush is meant only for the cheeks, this means do not apply your blush to your chin or forehead.

- Apply a light natural shade of blush to the cheekbones moving in an upward swirl to the hairline.

- Apply a brighter pink or peach just to the apples of the cheek then lightly blended into the natural shade to bring the two colors together. This will brighten your face for a realistic blushing bride finish.

- Do not overdo your blush application. You want your cheeks to have color but not look overdone.

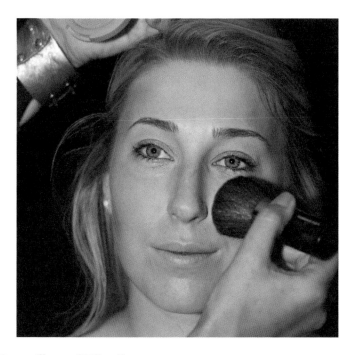

Benefits of Blush

Your blush can play an important role in your makeup routine if applied with care and precision. Your blush needs to be lightweight, the right color, and reflective, giving just the right amount of subtle glow to your face. When applied properly it will give the illusion of a woman who is ready to take on the day even if she might have had to little sleep the night before.

Step 7: Showcasing Your Eyes

Showcasing your eyes is the most challenging application of the entire makeup application but if you follow these easy to apply steps you will master the technique very quickly. Everyday makeup is not the time to have heavy smoky eyes or to test out trendy new looks. Your daily makeup is about an ethereal look that enhances your natural beauty. Avoid bright or dark colors, stick to pinks, peaches, light grays or charcoal.

Shadowing Steps

- Apply primer to the eyelids.

- Apply a light beige to the entire eye lid.

- Apply a pink or peach to the lower lid stopping at the crease line.

- Apply a charcoal or dark brown to the outer corner of the lower lid in the crease line, blending 1/3 of the way toward the center and then to the lash line 1/3 of the way in. Blend well.

- Apply a shimmer beige or light silver to the inner corner of the lower lid and just below the brow on the brow bone.

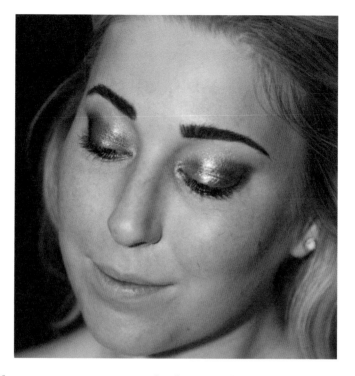

The secret to great eye shadow application is using quality products with a high pigment content, while at the same time using a quality brush that blends well to get seamlessness look of each color coming together with no lines of demarcation.

Showcasing your eyes is important, you want your eyes to look alluring and attractive, but try not to overdo the look, keep it simple and flawless.

Eye Liner

Eye liner doesn't have to be difficult it can be challenging at first to understand how to hold your brush and how to get a smooth line. Practicing everyday using quality brushes eye lining can be easy to achieve.

Try the tight lining technique for your eyeliner to showcase the eyes, this technique is much easier to apply using damp eye shadow and a liner brush or very fine gel eye liner pencil. Don't be afraid to test out liner products. This technique can be done with powder shadows, liner pencil or lose pigments.

- Line the upper lash line with a dark charcoal, dark brown or light black.
- Line the lower lash line with the same color coming in only 3/4 of the way.
- Soften the liner by smudging it with a bigger flat brush.

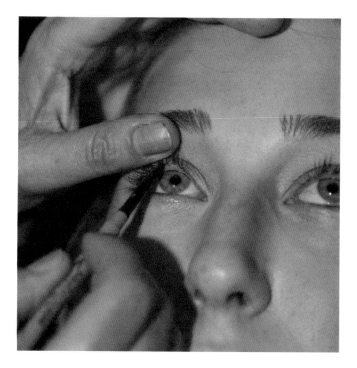

Eye lining is a skill that requires a lot of practice. The technique we used on our model is achieved by using a black eye shadow, we wet the brush with rose water to create a paste then applied the paste with a fine lining brush to the upper lash line and the lower lash line and to the upper inside lash line. You can darken the look be adding a gel liner over the top of the upper lash line when you have completed your entire eye makeup application.

Brows

Defining the eye brows will create a natural frame for the face and make eyes pop in photos. Be sure to use the correct color brow powder or brow pencil to fill-in brows, we suggest a two-color brow process to get a natural look.

- Apply the first color the same as your natural brow color or hair color to the lower brow line and move in hair like strokes to the outer brow line and follow it down to the tail.

- Use the lighter color to the inside corner of the brow using hair like strokes and to the upper hairline to give the brow depth and definition.

- You may also want to use a brow bone brightener under the brow bone to enhance the brow and make it stand out on the face.

It takes time to perfect a brow look and lots of practice. I suggest going to a pro makeup artist or skincare specialist to teach you this technique if you struggle with this application.

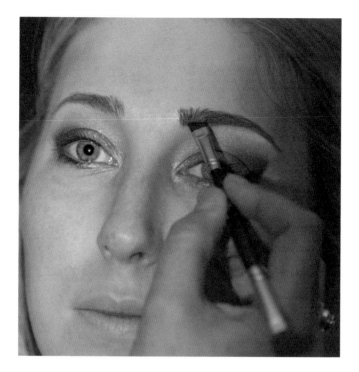

Your brows complete the face and without some type of enhancement or correction you can leave your face looking unfinished. Brow products come in pencils, powders and even gels.

Benefits of the Brow

Your brows may seem like the last thing you need to focus on during your makeup routine but even a small amount of brow shaping can make a huge difference in your completed makeup look.

Eye Brow Shaping

Eye brow shaping is a skill you will develop over time but the basic shape is as follows:

The brow starts on the inner corner of the nose.

Use a thin long brush or your eye brow pencil to gage the starting point of the brow. Place a small dot for you to start your brow line.

The arch of the brow should can be determined by holding your brow pencil at an angle coming up from the nose and running through the pupil on the eye.

Place a small dot to gage where the high point of the brow should be.

The outer corner of the brow can be determined by placing the brow pencil at a wide angle coming our from the corner of the nose and running on the outer corner of the eye. Place a small dot the gage where the eye brow should finish.

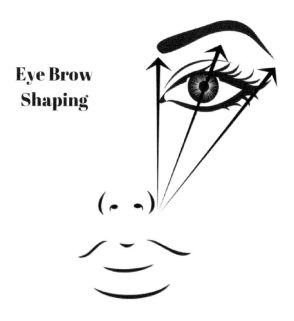

Eye Brow Shaping

Mascara

Enhancing your lashes will be the final step of your eye makeup application. Use a quality mascara that lengthens and plumps your lashes.

- Apply 1-3 coats till you have reached your desired length.
- Apply mascara starting in the middle of the lash and pulling upward and outward lengthening the lash to your desired fullness.

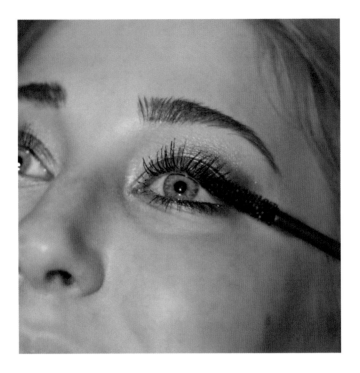

False Lashes

If you want more pop, the easiest false lash technique for a novice is to use individual lashes that come with three lashes on each band. These lashes can be applied to the outer 1/3 corner of your lash line after your mascara application. This is so much easier than learning to apply false lashes which can be a challenge for even the most qualified makeup artist. The last thing you want to happen on your wedding day is to have a lash strip come loose, this will mean pulling off both lash stripes leaving you without the long lush lashes you desire. You can get these individual lashes at any beauty supply store and even at high end retailers. Be sure to get the black glue used to apply the lashes so you don't have white dots on your lash line from the glue.

Lash Application

- Choose the length of lash you want to use.
- Apply the lash glue to the end of the lash.
- Wait one minute to let the glue setup.
- Apply the lash onto your lash line.
- Set the lash by pushing down on the tip of the lash until it blends with your own lashes.
- Apply the lashes to just the 1/3 outer corner of your lash line.
- Wait a few minutes for the lashes to firm up and dry into place.

Lashes are fun for special occasions but can look overdone for everyday wear. So I suggest you save the falsies for those special nights out on the town or when you are attending a special occasion.

Step 8: Lips

Lip sculpting has become the newest rage in makeup and although we do not recommend trend makeup in the everyday makeup application process we do think using this technique is a great way to give you the enhanced lips you are looking for. Achieving flawless lips is all about creating a plump and pouty look for a more romantic appearance to bring your lips forward and showcasing their beauty.

Your lip products will be the first makeup to disappear during the day so using our three step application will ensure a longer lasting look, but even with that said, make sure you have your daytime touch-up lip color on hand to refresh your look throughout the day. Carry your mini makeup kit to your purse in case you need to refresh your lips.

You will want to make sure you top off your lips right before you do any photo shoot. Use your lipstick throughout the day and keep it handy in an easy to access location.

When it comes to makeup your lips matter a great deal.

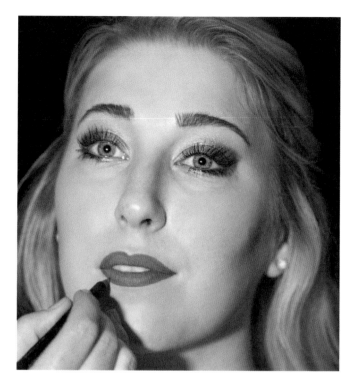

Lip Sculpting

- Line your lips with a color one shade darker than your natural lip color.

- Line the corners of your lips one third of the way in with the liner color.

- Fill in the area inside the lip liner with a shade that is exactly the same color as your natural lips with a lip liner pencil or lip stain.

- Top off your lips with a lipstick in pink, peach or plum or use your favorite lip gloss in a bright shade that pops to give your lips a lux look.

Natural lips with a pop of color are the secret to lip sculpting.

Starting with a natural base and building out the corners of the lips with a shade one color darker to give them definition, then topping your lips off with a blast of color and sealing it in with a gloss or lipstick to maintain it's longevity.

Lip Colors

Fair Skin: Nude, Pink, Mauve
Medium: Rose, Pink, Mauve
Olive: Peach, Coral, Dark Rose
Deep: Peach, Red, Coral

Choose the lip color you feel the most comfortable wearing and that fits into the appropriate time of the day. Not many women can pull off racing red lipstick during work hours but most women can pull of a true red for a night out on the town.

Step 9: Highlight & Brighten

Highlighting in a makeup application is a relatively new concept in everyday makeup but it has been a well kept secret of professional makeup artists. Makeup artists have been highlighting their clients for years and understand the importance of this step in the makeup application to brighten the face and get a pro finish. Makeup artists know the importance of highlighting to create more light on the face and to brighten up a flawless makeup application.

- Apply a powder highlighter below the brow, on the top of the brow bone, and on the top of your cheek bone over the top of your blusher.
- Apply your powder highlighter to the cupids bow on the top of your upper lip.
- Apply highlighter to your collarbone area after you have used bronzer to bring a subtle shimmer to your décolleté.

Try not to over highlight on the face. This can look tacky if it is a daytime makeup application and will create an over dramatic look on your face.

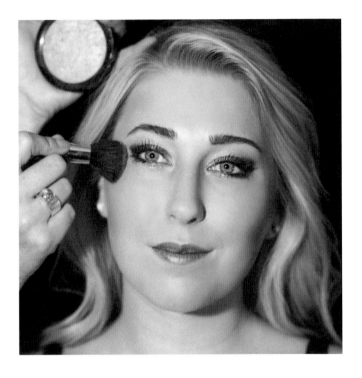

Highlighting your face at the end of your makeup application gives you a shimmering glamorous glow and will enhance any photo by giving the illusion of perfect lighting.

Step 10: Maintain Your Glow

The final step of success in your makeup look will be to keep your skin looking fresh and dewy all day, this will require diligence on your part throughout the day.

If you were unable to set your foundation and concealer with a setting powder you will now need to spritz your face with a setting spray.

Water

Hydration will be very important throughout the day to keep your skin plump and radiant. Dehydrated skin when left unattended will begin to appear sallow and will enhance fine lines, large pores, and wrinkles. To reduce the risk of appearing tired and to keep your makeup looking radiant it's best to keep well hydrated. Most women get so caught up in the business of the day that they tend to forget to keep their bodies hydrated.

Drinking water throughout the day and into the evening is the final step in keeping your gorgeous makeup looking flawless.

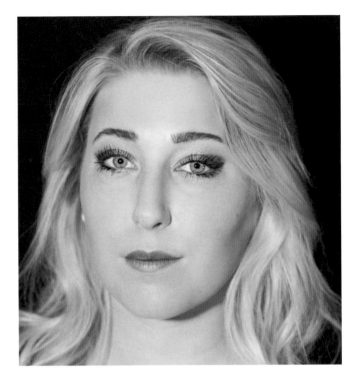

Setting Spray

Setting spray is the final step in your 10-step makeup application and one that I feel is very important to keep your makeup looking flawless all day. Spritz a very light spray of setting spray and wait for it to dry.

I encourage you to take time practicing your look until you have perfected it and you can apply it in less than 10 minutes.

Mature Makeup

Let's age beautifully.

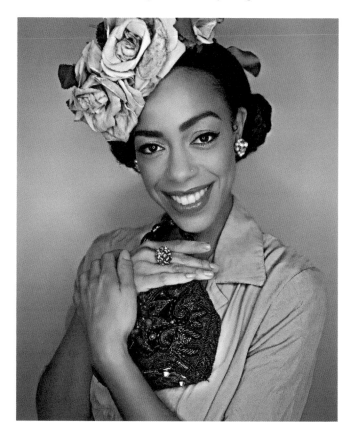

As women we often start wearing makeup when we are younger to help us look a bit older and as we age makeup continues to make us look older unless we reverse the rules we were taught when we were young. Makeup can look good on mature women if we apply a few new rules and use the products that enhance our skin to make it look fresh and glowing.

Prep

Before you can even begin your makeup application you will need to have well-prepared skin that is in tiptop condition. Exfoliation will improve the skin and its texture making your makeup application go on smoothly.

A good moisturizer will help to plump up the surface of the skin giving you a better canvas to work on. This means using a day cream as well as a good night cream along with a serum to keep the skin in the best condition. It will be up to you exfoliate and hydrate the skin at least once a week to help eliminate dead skin cells and promote new cell growth. You will want to be well hydrated before your makeup application with your recommended daily allowance of water.

Water is your skins best friend!

Less is More

This has never been truer than when working with mature skin. Less makeup really is the best approach while at the same time so is using the right products designed for your skin type and your mature skin.

Makeup

Prime: Using a face and eye primer is essential to a makeup application helping to minimize fine lines and pores as well as evening out skin tone and giving you the perfect base to lay down the makeup products.

Try to use a silicone-based primer if at all possible; this will give you the best coverage and foundation for the makeup you will apply.

Correct: As with other younger skin makeup applications you will have small issues to contend with on the face and it will be no different with mature skin. Often time's mature skin has hyper-pigmentation or age spots, as well as under eye darkness, for both of these issues use a lightweight creamy yellow toned corrector and dab it gently over the area working into the skin with your beauty blender or foundation brush. Let the corrector set for a few minutes before applying your foundation.

Broken capillaries are another issue with mature skin and must be dealt with before you apply your foundation. The best approach to this issue is to use a green-based corrector and gently dab the corrector into the skin with your blender or a brush. In both cases keep the amount of your corrector to a minimum and always give it time to settle in before applying your foundation.

Foundation: When we work with mature skin it is best to use a liquid foundation that is lightweight and reflective giving the skin a dewy look. Heavy cream foundations or powder foundations will only enhance fine lines and wrinkles, thus aging the skin and giving the appearance of covering the face instead of enhancing it. Use your foundation brush or beauty blender and gently buff the foundation on to the skin or dab it into the skin with a beauty blender. Never pull the skin with your brush or fingers you will only help to enhance fine lines with this technique.

Concealer: As with the foundation you want the under eye concealer to be liquid and light, be sure to use a concealer one shade lighter than your skin tone to brighten under the eyes and invoke youthfulness. Use your foundation brush or beauty blender and gently buff the foundation on to the skin or dab it into the skin.

Powder: Using a setting powder of foundation

powder on mature skin is not recommended. It will only enhance fine lines and pores and dull the skin making it look aged and flat.

Blush: Blush is the mature clients best friend, it will give a youthful glow promoting a healthy appearance. You can gently apply a light pink or peach blush to the apples of the cheeks then sweep it back to the temples. Once again use a light hand and layer the product to achieve the blush look you want to create. Do use a powder blush preferably with a little shimmer to it.

Eyes

As with your other makeup applications, the eyes will be the most challenging, the skin on mature eyes is very thin and often has a crêpe like texture. You may even find that mature eyes have become hooded and the floating lid invisible when the eyes are open. To overcome these issues you will want to make sure you have primed the eyes and avoid using heavy or dark shadow colors.

Eye Shadow: Find long-wearing shadows that are low in talc content and designed to prevent creasing on the eyelids. I recommend sticking with one color eye shadow in pink, peach, violet, or champagne and applying it to the floating lid and coming just above the crease line. Make sure you layer your shadow and blend it out so you don't have a harsh line of demarcation.

Eye Liner: Mature eyes are not always suitable for eyeliners but if you are used to wearing liner make sure you stay away from a black eye liner and use a brown or charcoal. I suggest a gel liner that you apply only to the top lash line or tight line on the top lash into the lashes, this will give your eyes depth and dimension and will be visible if you have hooded eyes.

Mascara: Mascara is essential for mature makeup and I suggest a dark brown shade that is not too harsh. Apply two or three coats of lengthening mascara to the lashes and focus on the outer corners to give the appearance of larger eyes. Hooded eyes can appear small in size and it is up to you to open up the face and bring attention to the eyes.

Brows: More often than not mature women have started to go gray in the brows and you will need to give the brows a boost with a brow product that looks natural and subtle.

I suggest using a cream brow product in taupe that you apply with a slanted brow brush and smudge it in with a spoolie. Less is more when it comes to brows but it is still important to do them to give symmetry to the face.

Lips

Mature lips have thinner skin and fine lines running out to the face. This happens when our skin starts to lose its collagen and wrinkles start to appear. To overcome this issue you will want to be very attentive to the lips and give them the love they need.

Lip Liner: Mature lips need a lip liner to stop the feathering of lipstick and lip-gloss so make sure you line the lips as well as use a concealer pencil around the edges of the lips to keep the product where it belongs. Apply the concealer from the bow of the lip all the way around the outside then blend into the skin. Apply the lip liner all the way around the lips.

Lipstick: Keep your lipstick subtle and light in color; dark lipsticks tend to make your client's lips look smaller and her face look older. Try pinks or peach based lipsticks and if she is used to dark colors choose a dark mauve to appease her. Top off the lips with a clear gloss or shimmer to give them a youthful glow. Using a lip brush will make the application smooth and crisp.

A mature woman can look just as radiant as younger women if you take the time to keep your makeup routine simple and apply the less is more concept. Stay away from heavy makeup and remember it is all about light and airy, dewy and glowing.

Lighting

All the cosmetics in the world will do us no good if we cant properly see to apply them. One of my top priorities, when I work with a client, is to encourage them to change out the vanity lights in their bathrooms to daylight light bulbs. This will help you to eliminate the yellow tones that regular light bulbs transmit and let you get better results when applying your makeup.

If you are having trouble seeing well to apply your makeup I suggest you find a quality tabletop lighted mirror that also has magnification to help you see as you apply products on your face.

Age is a wonderful thing when you embrace it and I believe we should all age beautifully.

Makeup Kit Checklist
The basics for your beauty arsenal.

Often all we need are a few added items to our makeup collection to create the ultimate makeup magic makeup kit. You may only need a few of the items listed to complete your kit or you might want to start from the beginning. Either way here is our essential makeup magic kit list.

Primer – Lightweight and suited for your skin type.

Corrector – Only if needed to correct flaws.

Concealer – Lightweight and creamy that can cover as well as brighten under the eyes.

Foundation – A formula well suited to your skin type and perfectly matched to your skin tone.

Setting Powder – A translucent powder used as a light dusting to set your makeup and control shine.

Contour/Bronzer – One shade darker than your skin tone to sculpt the face.

Blush – Pink, peach, or plum in a warm tone to bring a hint of color to the face.

3 Color Shadow Palette – One that contains a neutral shade, a medium shade, and a rich shade to create the perfect shadow look.

Eye Liner – Choose black for rich skin and dark brown for fair skin, used to define the outer edges of the eyes.

Mascara – Your favorite formula created to define the eyes and enhance the lashes.

Brow Product – Complete your eye look by defining the brows in your favorite powder, pot, or pencil formula.

Lip Pencil – Used to define the lips and keep the lipstick in place all day. Use a natural lip color that matches your lips.

Lipstick – Lipstick or a lip gloss in your favorite color. Be sure to choose the right colors for your skin tone.

Highlighter – A little shimmer can go a long way and isn't always needed for a daytime look, but it's perfect for a night out.

Setting Spray – The lightweight spray that will hold your makeup in place for the long run.

Quality Brushes – A complete set of face and eye brushes to apply your makeup and get a flawless finish.

Tweezers – To help you apply false lashes and pluck those stray brow hairs between brow appointments.

Makeup Bag – A quality and durable bag to carry all your makeup and keep it all in one convenient location.

Makeup Mirror – Good lighting to help you get a great makeup application every time.

Resources

Finding quality makeup is not always easy and honestly, with so many choices, it can frankly be overwhelming. Just step into a Sephora store if you don't know what I'm talking about. Overwhelming is an understatement.

I have decided to add this small section in the book to help you in your search for quality makeup and tools that you don't even need to leave your house for.

Please note these products are just a few that I like and feel qualified to share with you, online shopping can also be overwhelming, so make a list of what you need, and stick to only buying only the cosmetic products you need or know and trust. Not all makeup works with every skin tone or skin type so you decide which brands work best for you. Do your research before you begin and then do all you can to keep your makeup routine simple, easy, and flawless.

Remember getting the right color foundation for your skin is a critical step in your makeup routine and may require that you seek a consultation with a specialist to get an exact match for your skin tone and skin type. You might also want to take a Mother-Daughter Day or Friends Out on the Town Day and get mini makeovers at a few of your local cosmetics counters or from a qualified makeup artist who offers this service.

Getting the right products will take time and dedication to yourself but isn't your face worth it?

Suggested Books on Makeup

Bobbi Brown Makeup Manual (Bobbi Brown)

Face Forward (Kevyn Aucoin)

DIY Bridal Makeup (Toni Thomas & Keisha Garrett)

Suggested Cosmetic Companies

Mally Cosmetics ~ mallycosmetics.com

E.L.F. Cosmetics ~ elfcosmetics.com

Bobbi Brown ~ bobbibrowncosmetics.com

NARS Cosmetics ~ narscosmetics.com

BH Cosmetics ~ bhcosmetics.com

Benefit Cosmetics ~ benefitcosmetics.com

NYX Cosmetics ~ nyxcosmetics.com

Morphe Brushes ~ morphebrushes.com

Riki Mirror ~ glamcor.com

The list for quality cosmetics could go on forever and would take up hundreds of pages. It will be up to you to find the products that work best for you and your certain cosmetic needs.

You choose the brand and products you like and take the time to get mini makeovers from qualified professionals who can assist you in your search for the products that work best for you.

ABOUT THE AUTHOR

Toni Thomas is an award-winning beauty industry professional, makeup artist, beauty educator, and author of several beauty industry books. Her makeup artistry has been seen on the runway at New York Fashion Week, in editorial publications, and on the faces of many women. She is the founder of Women in Gear, School of Makeup Artistry an online education portal for aspiring makeup artists. Toni has spent her entire career in the beauty industry working in and around the beauty and fashion business as well as the beauty education arena where she has taught for many years. Teaching in the world of beauty to those who are willing to take a leap of faith on themselves is what she aspires to do the rest of her life. Her passion to inspire those who wish to pursue their dreams has made a global impact on the world of business, makeup artistry, and beauty.

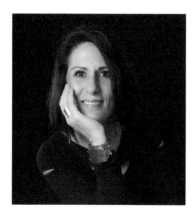

Printed in Great Britain
by Amazon